Understanding
Chemotherapy

BACUP 121-123 Charterhouse Street, London, EC1M 6AA

BACUP was founded by Dr Vicky Clement-Jones, following her own experiences with ovarian cancer, and offers information, advice and emotional support to cancer patients and their families.

We produce publications on the main types of cancer, treatments, and ways of living with cancer. We also produce a newspaper, *BACUP News*, three times a year.

Our success depends on feedback from users of the service. We thank everyone, particularly patients and their families, whose advice has made this booklet possible.

Administration 071 608 1785   Charity Registration No. 290526
Cancer Information Service 071 608 1661 (6 lines)
Freeline (outside London) 0800 181199
Counselling Service 071 608 1038 (London based)

Editor: Dr Maurice Slevin, MD, FRCP

Deputy Editor: Patsy Ryan, RGN

Publications Consultant: Elizabeth Sturgeon

Design: Rosie Cleghorn

Cover illustration by Malcolm Harvey Young

Text illustrations by Alexa Rutherford

We gratefully acknowledge Sally Openshaw SRN for her help with this booklet.

Typeset and printed in Great Britain by Lithoflow Ltd., London

ISBN 1-870403-38-X

Contents

Introduction

This information booklet has been written to help you, your family and friends understand more about chemotherapy. We hope it answers some of the questions you may have about this type of cancer treatment and how to cope with any side effects it may produce.

The information on chemotherapy is divided into sections on how the treatment works, how it is given and how to manage some of the more common possible side effects. Although this booklet can help you to understand what happens during chemotherapy treatment, you are still likely to have more questions and concerns about your own treatment. As there are over 200 different types of cancer and many variations of chemotherapy treatment it is best to discuss specific details of your own treatment with your doctor.

At the end of the booklet, there is a list of other BACUP publications, some useful addresses and recommended books. If, after reading this booklet, you think it has helped you, do pass it on to any of your family and friends who may find it interesting. They too may want to be informed so they can help you cope with any problems you may have.

What is chemotherapy?

The type of treatment you are given for your cancer depends on many factors, particularly the type of cancer you have, where in the body it started, what the cancer cells look like under the microscope and how far they have spread, if at all.

Chemotherapy is the use of anti-cancer (cytotoxic) drugs to destroy cancer cells. The word simply means drug treatment and it is taken from two words — 'chemical' and 'therapy'. Chemotherapy treatment can be just one drug or several drugs, taken from a choice of about 40 different drugs available.

Chemotherapy may be used alone to treat cancer or together with surgery and/or radiotherapy.

How do the drugs work ?

Cancer is a disease of the body's cells. Normally, all cells divide and reproduce themselves in an orderly and controlled manner. In cancer, however, the process gets out of control and the cells multiply without proper control, forming a lump (which is called a tumour) or in leukaemia, producing too many white blood cells.

Sometimes cancer cells break away from a tumour and travel to other parts of the body via the bloodstream or lymphatic system. (The lymphatic system is a network of fine channels – called lymph vessels – which run throughout the body). When the cancer cells reach other parts of the body they may settle and start to develop into new tumours. These are known as secondary cancers or metastases.

Chemotherapy drugs work by interfering with the ability of a cancer cell to divide and reproduce itself. The affected cells become damaged and eventually die. As the drugs are carried in the blood, they can reach cancer cells all over the body.

The drugs damage the cancer cells in different ways. If a combination of drugs is used, each drug is chosen because of its different effects. Unfortunately, chemotherapy drugs can also affect normal cells in your body, sometimes causing unpleasant side effects. Unlike cancer cells, however, normal cells quickly regrow, so any damage to them is usually temporary and therefore most side effects will disappear once the treatment is over.

The cure rates vary from the majority in some cancers to the minority in others, depending on the type of cancer. In some cancers, cure may be less likely and then chemotherapy may be given to shrink the cancer, prolong life and relieve symptoms.

How are the drugs given?

Chemotherapy may be given by a number of different routes, depending on the type of cancer you have and the drugs used. The most usual ways are by mouth (orally) or injection into a vein (intravenously). Less commonly used ways are by injection into a muscle (intramuscularly) or under the skin (subcutaneously). Sometimes, two or more routes may be used together. Whichever way the drugs are given, they are absorbed into the blood and carried around the body so they can reach all the cancer cells.

Giving the drugs by mouth

You may be given tablets to take at home as all or part of your treatment. You will be told when to take them and given other specific instructions such as whether or not to take them with food. If, for any reason, you cannot take your tablets as prescribed you should contact your doctor immediately for advice.

Giving the drugs by intravenous injection

Sometimes the drugs are diluted into a large volume of liquid and given via a 'drip' into a vein in your arm. In these cases, a fine tube will be inserted into the vein and taped securely to your arm. This tube is called a cannula.

The other way of giving intravenous chemotherapy is via a plastic line (called a central line) put into a vein in your chest. A Hickman line is one type commonly used. Unlike the cannula used for the vein in an arm, a central line is inserted after you have been given a general or local anaesthetic. Once it is in place, the central line is either stitched or taped firmly to your chest to prevent it being pulled out of the vein. It can remain in the vein for many months and means you will not need to have needles when you have your intravenous chemotherapy. Blood for testing can also be taken via this line. It has to be kept extremely clean to prevent an infection getting into the bloodstream, so it needs to be flushed daily with sterile water. The nurses on the ward will teach you how to do this yourself.

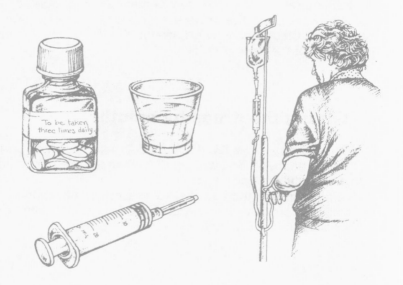

Intravenous chemotherapy drugs are given over a period of time, usually ranging from half an hour to a few hours, or sometimes a few days. If it only takes a few hours, the drugs can be given to you as an outpatient at the hospital. If a few days are needed, you will be admitted to a ward at the hospital.

Some chemotherapy drugs can be put into electric pumps that give a controlled amount of the drug into the bloodstream over a specified period of time. These pumps are portable and after they have been set up in the outpatients department, you can go home with them.

Where is the treatment given

Some chemotherapy drugs can be given to you as an outpatient at the hospital but other chemotherapy treatments will mean a short stay in hospital – perhaps overnight or for a couple of days. Occasionally chemotherapy treatments will mean you need to stay in hospital for longer; perhaps a few weeks. Your doctor will be happy to explain exactly what your treatment will involve before it starts.

Treatment planning

Your doctor will take several factors into consideration when planning your treatment. The most important of these are the type of cancer you have, where in the body it is situated and how far it has spread, if at all. Other factors include your age and general health. This means you will find other patients at the hospital are having different chemotherapy.

The frequency of your treatment and the length of time it takes will depend on several factors including: the type of cancer you have, the drugs you are taking, the response of the cancer cells to the drugs and any side effects the drugs may cause.

Chemotherapy is usually given as several courses of treatment. Depending on the drug or drugs given, each course can last from a few hours to a few days. Each course is followed by a rest period of a few weeks which allows your body to recover from any side effects of the treatment. The total number of courses you have will depend on how well your cancer is responding to the drugs. It may take several months to complete all the chemotherapy courses needed for the treatment of your cancer. Some patients on oral chemotherapy take smaller doses of chemotherapy daily for several weeks or months, before they have a rest period.

It may be necessary for you to have blood tests or X-rays, or to see the doctor before you are given your chemotherapy and this will obviously all take time. All chemotherapy drugs are prepared in a special way and you may have to wait while the hospital pharmacy department prepares them to dispense to you. To help pass the time, it can be helpful to take a book, newspaper, crosswords or perhaps some letters to write.

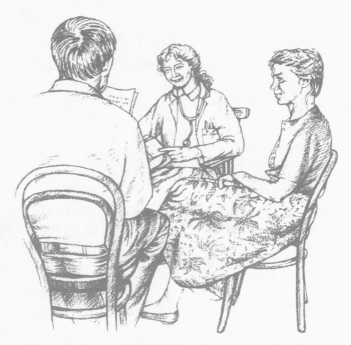

Your doctor will be happy to explain your own treatment plan to you and if you have any questions don't be afraid to ask your doctor or ward sister. It often helps to make a list of questions for your doctor and to take a close relative or friend with you to remind you of things you want to know but can so easily forget.

Changes in the treatment plan

Your doctor will be assessing regularly the effects of the chemotherapy on your cancer. In order to do this you may need frequent blood tests, X–rays and scans. The results from these tests show the doctor how much the cancer is reducing in size in response to the treatment. Sometimes, depending on the results of the tests, your treatment plan may need to be modified in some way or even changed completely. Sometimes this is because the present drugs you are having are not shrinking the cancer sufficiently and changing to different drugs may produce a more effective reponse. Occasionally, your treatment may also be delayed because the chemotherapy drugs are preventing your bone marrow from functioning properly (see page 18). Delaying the chemotherapy gives your bone marrow a chance to recover before the next course of drugs is given.

Treatment can also sometimes be delayed to fit in with special occasions you wish to attend and it is sometimes possible to arrange your treatment around your holiday dates.

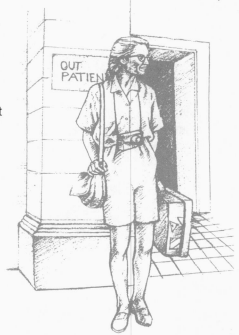

What are the side effects of chemotherapy?

Not everyone being treated with chemotherapy will have side effects. Cancer treatments produce different reactions in different people and any reaction can vary from treatment to treatment. It may be helpful to remember that almost all side effects are only temporary and will gradually disappear once the treatment has stopped.

The main areas of your body that may be particularly affected by chemotherapy are those where normal cells rapidly divide and grow, such as your mouth, digestive system, skin, hair and bone marrow (the spongy material that fills the bones and produces new blood cells).

If you want to know more about specific side effects which may be caused by your own chemotherapy treatment you should ask your doctor, as he or she will know the exact drugs you are taking. Although the side effects of chemotherapy can be unpleasant, they must be weighed against the benefits of the treatment. If, however, you are finding the treatment or its side effects are making you unwell, do tell your doctor, who may be able to give you medicines to help, or make changes to your treatment to lessen any side effects.

If you would like to talk to one of the nurses at BACUP they will be happy to help.

Possible side effects of some chemotherapy drugs

Your mouth

Some chemotherapy drugs can cause a sore mouth and, sometimes, small mouth ulcers. If this is going to happen it usually occurs about five to ten days after the drugs are given and will clear up within three to four weeks. Sometimes the mouth ulcers can become infected. If this does happen, your doctor can give you treatment to help clear infection.

Some chemotherapy drugs can cause your taste to change; food may taste more salty, bitter or metallic. Normal taste will return once the chemotherapy treatment is over.

Helpful hints

■ Clean your mouth and teeth gently every morning, evening and after each meal.

■ A soft – bristled or child's toothbrush will be kinder to a sore mouth.

■ Remove and clean dentures every morning, evening and after each meal.

■ If your toothpaste stings, or brushing your teeth makes you feel nauseous, try a bicarbonate of soda mouthwash instead. (One teaspoon of bicarbonate of soda dissolved in a mug of warm water.)

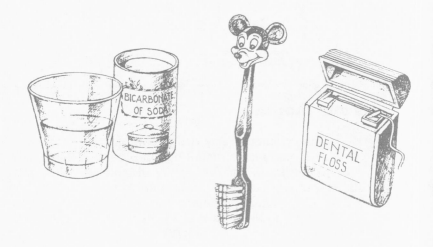

■ Use dental floss daily.

■ Keep your lips moist by using Vaseline or a flavoured lip balm if you prefer.

■ Avoid neat spirits, tobacco, hot spices, garlic, onion, vinegar and salty food. These may increase abnormal tastes and irritate your mouth.

■ Keep your mouth and food moist. Add gravies and sauces to your food to make swallowing easier and try to drink at least one and a half litres (three pints) of fluid a day, in the form of beverages (tea or coffee), fruit and vegetable juices and soft drinks.

■ Let your doctor know if you develop mouth ulcers, as you may need drug treatment to help heal the ulcers and prevent or clear any mouth infection.

Your digestive system

Sickness is a side effect associated with some chemotherapy drugs. Many people do not have any nausea and vomiting with their chemotherapy, nor does every drug cause sickness. If you are affected, however, the sickness will start from a few minutes to several hours after chemotherapy injections, depending on the drugs given. The sickness may last for a few hours and occasionally you may continue to feel sick the next day. In rare cases, the sickness may continue for several days. There are, however, several anti-sickness drugs (antiemetics) which your doctor can prescribe to help relieve your sickness.

This sick feeling may cause you to lose your appetite for a time. Your appetite may also be affected by the changes in taste sometimes caused by chemotherapy treatment. These changes may mean you go off certain types of food or that some foods will taste different from usual. Some patients have an abnormal taste in their mouths during their chemotherapy treatment (see the section on 'Your mouth')

The lining of the digestive system may be affected by some chemotherapy drugs and this may cause diarrhoea. If this is going to happen, frequent loose stools may be passed in the first few days following chemotherapy. More rarely, some chemotherapy drugs can cause constipation. If you do have any changes in your bowel habits, it is advisable to inform your doctor.

Helpful hints

■ **If you do have nausea and vomiting it is very important to tell your doctor as soon as possible. He or she can prescribe anti-sickness drugs for you (antiemetics) which are usually very effective.**

■ Avoid eating or preparing food when you feel nauseous.

■ Avoid fried foods, fatty foods or foods with a strong odour.

■ Eat cold or slightly warm food if the smell of cooked or cooking food causes nausea.

■ Eat several small meals and snacks each day and chew the food well.

■ Do not eat directly before treatment, but do have a small meal a few hours earlier.

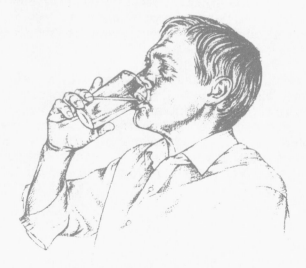

■ Drink plenty of liquid, slowly, taking small sips. Avoid filling your stomach with a large volume of water before eating.

- If you do have diarrhoea, eat less fibre, avoiding raw fruits, cereals and vegetables. Avoid the foods mentioned earlier which can irritate the mouth and alter taste.

- Drink plenty of liquid to replace the fluid lost in diarrhoea.

- If constipation occurs, increase your intake of fibre, raw fruits, cereals, fluids and vegetables. Prune juice and hot drinks can often stimulate bowel action.

- Eating fresh pineapple chunks helps to keep your mouth fresh and moist.

- Some people find that using relaxation techniques helps to fend off or lessen their nausea. The BACUP nurses have lists of tapes, books and classes which teach these techniques.

If you are worried about the effects of chemotherapy on your digestive system, it is important to see your doctor and discuss any problems you may have coping with these side effects. BACUP has a booklet called "Diet and the Cancer Patient" with plenty of tips on how to eat well when you feel ill.

Your hair and skin

Hair loss is one of the most well-known side effects of chemotherapy. Some chemotherapy drugs cause no hair loss or the amount of hair lost is so slight it is hardly noticeable. Others, however, do cause temporary partial or complete baldness. Some chemotherapy drugs can damage hair, causing it to break off at or near the scalp a week or two after the chemotherapy has started. The amount of hair lost, if any, depends on the type of drug or combination of drugs used, the dosage given and the person's individual reaction to the drug.

If hair loss is going to occur, it usually starts within a few weeks of beginning treatment, although very occasionally it can start within a few days. Body and pubic hair may be lost as well. **If you do lose your hair as a result of chemotherapy, it will always grow back once you have completed your treatment.**

Some chemotherapy drugs can affect your skin. The drugs may cause your skin to become dry, slightly discoloured or more sensitive to sunlight. Any rashes should be reported to your doctor. Your nails may grow more slowly and you may notice white ridges appearing across them.

Helpful hints

- If your drugs are likely to cause hair loss, consider having your hair cut quite short prior to treatment. The weight of long hair pulls on the scalp and may increase the rate of hair loss if it is going to occur.

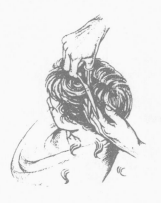

- Use gentle hair products and avoid the harsh chemicals found in perms and hair colourings.

- Try not to brush or comb your hair too vigorously – a soft baby brush may help.

- Avoid using hair driers, curling tongs and curlers. Gently patting hair dry will be less harmful.

- If it is likely you may lose your hair, ask your doctor about wigs early on, so the wig can be as close a match as possible to the colour and texture of your real hair. There are many other ways of disguising hair loss and these are discussed in BACUP's 'Coping With Hair Loss' booklet.

- If your skin becomes dry or itchy, rubbing in a little lanolin cream can help to relieve it.

- False nails or nail varnish can be used to disguise split and ridged nails.

- Wear a high factor sun-blocking cream if you are going out in the sun, to prevent your skin burning.

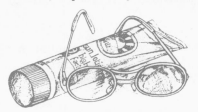

Some people having certain chemotherapy drugs may be able to prevent hair loss by using a "cold cap". This works by temporarily narrowing the blood vessels of the scalp, decreasing the amount of chemotherapy drug reaching the hair follicles (the cells from which hair grows). Unfortunately, the cold cap does not work for everyone as it only blocks the action of certain chemotherapy drugs. It is best to ask your doctor whether one would be useful in your case.

BACUP has a booklet called 'Coping With Hair Loss' which we would be happy to send you.

Your bone marrow

B one marrow is a spongy material that fills the bones and contains cells which normally develop into the three different types of blood cell.

■ **Red blood cells contain haemoglobin to carry oxygen around the body:**

If the level of haemoglobin in your blood is low you will become very tired and lethargic. Because the amount of oxygen being carried around your body is decreased, you may also become breathless. These are all symptoms of anaemia – a lack of haemoglobin in the blood.

Anaemia is very successfully treated by blood transfusions. The extra red cells in the blood transfusion will very quickly pick up the oxygen from your lungs and transport it around the body to other tissues and organs. You will feel more energetic and the breathlessness will be eased.

During your chemotherapy treatment you will have regular blood tests to count the number of red cells in the blood and will be given blood transfusions each time you are running short of these cells.

■ **White blood cells are essential for fighting infections:**

If the number of white cells in your blood is low you will be more prone to infection as there are fewer white cells to fight off bacteria and viruses.

As white blood cells are the body's most important line of defence against infection you may be given antibiotics during your chemotherapy treatment to help them fight off any infections. Your regular blood tests will also calculate the number of white cells in the blood and you may need antibiotics given directly into the blood (intravenously) if your white cell count is low. Sometimes you may need to be admitted to hospital for antibiotic treatment.

■ **Platelets which help to clot the blood to prevent bleeding:**

If the number of platelets in your blood is low you will bruise very easily and may bleed heavily from even minor cuts or grazes; so if your platelet count is low you will need to be admitted to hospital for a platelet transfusion. This is similar to a blood transfusion but all the red cells and white cells have been removed and a clear fluid containing only platelets is transfused into your blood. These platelets will start to work immediately, clotting together to prevent bruising and bleeding as soon as the body is injured.

Your regular blood tests will also be used to count the number of platelets in your blood and you can have a platelet transfusion in hospital as often as necessary.

Helpful hints

■ **Inform your doctor IMMEDIATELY if you develop a fever (temperature over 38C) or notice any sign of bleeding or bruising while you are having chemotherapy or in the rest period after the treatment. These signs may indicate that your bone marrow is being affected by the chemotherapy.**

■ Try to avoid crowded places and people with infectious illness, but it is not necessary to become a hermit!

■ Maintain high standards of personal hygiene. Always wash your hands thoroughly before preparing your food.

■ Try to eat as healthy a diet as possible; include plenty of fresh fruit and salads. Ensure all your food is well cooked and avoid 'take aways'. BACUP's booklet "Diet and the Cancer Patient" has tips on how to eat healthily if you are feeling below par.

■ Take care to avoid injury if you are gardening – wear thick gloves.

■ Keep away from animals, especially their excreta (cat litter trays, bird cages)

■ If you do cut yourself at any time, you may need to apply pressure to the cut for longer than usual to stop the bleeding.

■ Rest whenever you feel tired. Try to avoid organising busy periods on the day of your treatment and take it easy for a couple of days afterwards.

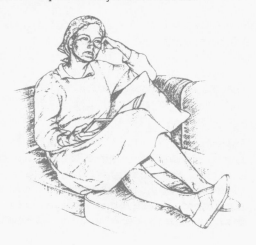

Will chemotherapy affect my everyday life?

E
ven though chemotherapy treatment can cause unpleasant side effects, some people still manage to lead an almost normal life during their treatment. Even if you feel unwell during your treatment course, many people find they recover quickly between courses and can resume their usual activities as they begin to feel better. If you are taking chemotherapy tablets at home, you may find the treatment causes very little disruption to your everyday life. If you are having oral chemotherapy, depending on how you feel, you may still be able to go to work and carry on with your social activities as usual.

Some intravenous chemotherapy can be given to you as an outpatient at the hospital, but if you do need to spend time in hospital, you are likely to need to make more changes to your usual routines. Most employers will be sympathetic if you explain why you need time off work. If you are unable to work, your employer will pay your first 28 weeks' sick pay. If, after this period, you are still unable to work you can claim Invalidity Benefit from the DSS.

If you are unemployed and not fit to work you will need to switch from Unemployment Benefit to Sickness Benefit. To do this you should contact your local DSS office and arrange to send regular sickness certificates from your doctor.

Social workers at the hospital or attached to your family doctor's surgery can help you find out about any benefits or social services to which you are entitled while you are having chemotherapy. Your local Citizens' Advice Bureau can also give useful information and advice on available benefits.

During intravenous chemotherapy you may find you cannot do some of the things you used to take for granted, but you needn't abandon your social life completely. Depending on how well you feel, there is no reason to stop going out or visiting friends, especially if you can plan ahead for social occasions. For example, if you are going out for the evening, you could make sure you get plenty of rest during the day so you have more energy for the evening. If you are planning to go out for a meal, you may find it helpful to take anti-sickness tablets before you go and to choose your food carefully from the menu.

For most people, having the occasional alcoholic drink will not affect their chemotherapy treatment.

If you are going abroad on holiday, it is extremely important to remember that you should not have any 'live virus' vaccines while you are having chemotherapy. These include polio, measles, rubella (German Measles), MMR (the new triple vaccine for measles, mumps and rubella), BCG (tuberculosis) and yellow fever. There are, however, vaccines which you can have, if necessary, while you are having chemotherapy. These include whooping cough, diptheria, tetanus, 'flu, hepatitis B, rabies, cholera, typhoid and anthrax.

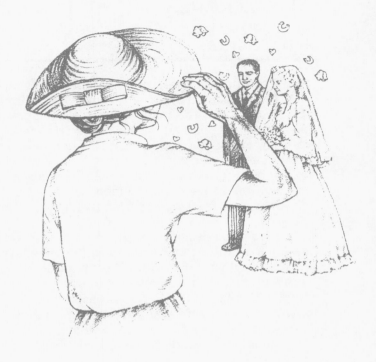

If you have a really important social event coming up,
discuss with your doctor whether your treatment can be
altered so that you can feel as well as possible for the
occasion.

Will chemotherapy make me infertile ?

Not all chemotherapy treatment causes infertility but unfortunately there are some chemotherapy drugs which do. The infertility may be temporary or permanent, depending on the drugs you are having. It is very important that you discuss this risk fully with your doctor before you start treatment. Your partner will probably be anxious to join you at this discussion so you can both be aware of all the facts and have a chance to talk over your feelings and options for the future.

It is quite possible for a woman having chemotherapy, or the female partner of a man having chemotherapy, to become pregnant during the treatment. Pregnancy should be avoided during chemotherapy, however, in case the drugs affect the baby. For this reason, your doctor will advise you to ensure you use a reliable method of contraception (usually "barrier" methods of contraception – such as condoms or the cap) throughout your treatment.

For women:

Although not all chemotherapy drugs will cause you to become infertile, some may affect your ovaries and stop them producing eggs which can be fertilised by the male sperm during sex. If this does happen it means, unfortunately, that you can no longer become pregnant and it will also bring on symptoms normally associated with going through the 'change of life' (the menopause). Your monthly periods may become irregular and eventually stop completely and you may experience 'hot flushes', dry skin and dryness of the vagina.

Depending on the type of cancer you have, your doctor can often prescribe hormone tablets for you to take before your chemotherapy treatment starts, to help prevent these side effects. The hormones, unfortunately, will not enable you to start producing eggs again and so cannot prevent infertility. Your doctor or nurse may also suggest a cream or ointment which you can get on prescription or buy from the chemist which can moisten the vagina and help to make sex more comfortable.

If the infertility is temporary; that is, your ovaries are going to start producing eggs again, your periods will return to normal once your treatment has finished. This does happen in about a third of all previously fertile women who were made temporarily infertile by their chemotherapy treatment.

If you are pregnant before your cancer is diagnosed and your chemotherapy starts, it is extremely important to discuss fully with your doctor the pros and cons of continuing with your pregnancy. It is occasionally possible to delay starting chemotherapy treatment until after the baby is born, but this is a rare situation and depends largely on the type of cancer you have and the extent of the disease, as well as the drugs you will be taking. You will need to talk to your doctor very frankly about your pregnancy and be sure you are fully aware of all the risks and alternatives before making any decisions.

For men

Some chemotherapy drugs will have no effect at all on your fertility, but others may reduce the number of sperm you produce or affect their ability to reach and fertilise a female egg during sex. Unfortunately, this means you may no longer be able to father children. You will still, however, be able to get an erection and orgasm as you did before you started your treatment. No chemotherapy drugs will have any permanent effect whatsoever on your sexual performance or your ability to enjoy sex.

If you have not completed your family before you need to start chemotherapy treatment, you may be able to bank some of your sperm for later use. If this is possible in your case, you will be asked to produce several sperm samples over a few weeks. These will then be frozen and stored. If you and your partner later want a baby, the samples can be thawed and used to inseminate your partner artificially. The pregnancy should then carry on as normal.

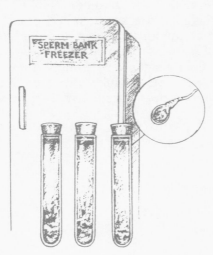

If the chemotherapy did cause infertility, after their treatment has stopped some men will remain infertile, while a few find their sperm returns to normal and their fertility is restored. Your doctor will be able to do a sperm count for you when your treatment is over to check your fertility.

Teenage boys should also be aware of the infertility risk so that, if possible, their sperm can be stored for later years.

Your feelings

Many people are devastated when they discover that the treatment they need to help beat their cancer will also mean they can no longer have any children. Infertility is very hard to come to terms with, especially if you were planning to have children in the future or to have more children to complete your family. The sense of loss can be acute for people of all ages. Sometimes it can feel as though you have actually lost a part of yourself. You may feel less manly or less feminine because you can't have children. Women especially may be distressed and resentful that the drugs may cause bodily changes (like the menopause) which undermine their self-confidence even further.

Obviously, people vary in their reactions to the risk of infertility. Some people may seem to shrug it off and feel that beating the cancer is more important. Others may seem to accept the news calmly when they start treatment and find that the true impact doesn't hit them until the treatment is over and they are picking up the pieces of their lives again.

There is no right or wrong way to react. Each person is individual and reactions will depend on different circumstances and ambitions. What is important is that you discuss with your doctor the risks and all your options fully before you start treatment, and that you have an opportunity to talk over any emotions which threaten to get too much for you, with a trained counsellor if necessary.

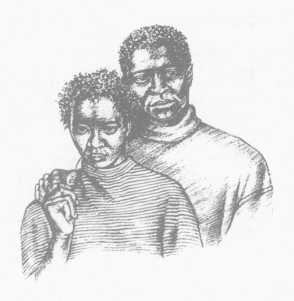

Your partner will also need special consideration in any discussions about fertility and future plans. You may find that you both need to speak to a professional counsellor or therapist specialising in fertility problems, in order to start coming to terms with your situation.

Your doctor may be able to refer you to a specialist or you can be put in touch directly with one by contacting the organisations listed at the back of this booklet. The nurses at the BACUP cancer information service are always very willing to discuss problems you may have of any nature and they can also put you in touch with counsellors throughout the country who can offer you help and advice. BACUP has its own counselling service, available by appointment at its London offices.

Will chemotherapy affect my sex life?

M any people go through their chemotherapy with their usual sex lives unaffected. On the other hand, some people may find their sex lives temporarily change in some way during their treatment.

Any changes that may occur, however, are usually simple and shortlived and should not have a long term effect on your sex life. For example, there may be times when you just feel too tired, or perhaps not strong enough to maintain the level of physical activity you are used to during sex. If your treatment is making you feel sick, you may go off sex altogether for a while. Anxiety may also play a large part in putting you off sex. Often this anxiety may not seem directly related to sex; you may be worried about your chances of surviving your cancer, or how your family are coping with the illness, or about your finances, but stresses like these can easily push everything else, including sex, to the back of your mind.

Any such changes are usually shortlived and not serious. The most important thing to remember is that there is no medical reason whatsoever to stop having sex at any time during your chemotherapy course. It is perfectly safe to continue to enjoy sex and the chemotherapy drugs themselves will have no long term physical effects on your performance or ability to enjoy sex, nor will they affect your partner, apart from the increased need for adequate contraception.

The only exception may be women whose chemotherapy has brought on an early menopause (See page 24 on Fertility). These women will experience symptoms usually associated with the menopause, which may include dryness of the vagina and a decreased interest in sex (loss of libido). In many cases, depending on the type of cancer, your doctor can prescribe hormone replacement therapy (HRT) to prevent these symptoms (unfortunately, the HRT will not prevent the menopause). If dryness of the vagina is making sex uncomfortable, your doctor may be able to prescribe a cream or ointment to ease the problem, or you can use KY Jelly or other commercial preparations (available from your chemist without a prescription) to moisten the vagina.

If you are anxious that the chemotherapy could affect your sex life, try to discuss your worries with your doctor before your treatment starts – if you find him or her approachable enough to discuss personal matters without too much embarrassment. Your doctor should be able to tell you what, in general, are the side effects to expect from your treatment and you can then talk over the main implications of these, if any, on your sex life. Try not to feel embarrassed asking your doctor about possible sexual problems. You need to know about all aspects of your treatment, and if sex is an important part of your life, it matters that you should be fully aware of any possible changes.

Obviously, it may help if you can discuss your feelings and any worries with your partner. Even though it is unlikely you will have any problems with sex, your partner may still have some anxieties and may have been waiting for a cue from you to show that it is all right to discuss them. Perhaps your partner could join you if you decide you want to talk to your doctor. That way if either of you does have any worries, both your minds can be put at rest.

Trying to overcome any problem, sexual or otherwise, may seem like an uphill struggle when you are also trying to come to terms with your cancer and cope with chemotherapy. You may find it encouraging to know that any side effects from chemotherapy, such as tiredness or sickness, that may affect your sex life are only temporary (for some women the early menopause side effect is also temporary – see page 24) and will gradually wear off once your treatment is finished. You will then be free to carry on with your usual sex life as before.

How will I feel during chemotherapy?

Many people find that having cancer, needing chemotherapy treatment and the effect that both of these may have on their lives can sometimes make them feel anxious, afraid or depressed. Often these feelings can be prompted by something seemingly trivial, such as having to change your usual daily routine to fit in with the treatments, or something more obvious, such as the side effects of the treatment, or the risk of infertility. If you do feel low or worried, for whatever reason, it is important to know that you are not alone. You can be sure many cancer patients have felt as you do at some time during their treatment and that, like them, you can overcome feeling fearful or discouraged.

One of the first steps to solving problems successfully is to identify exactly what is causing the problem in the first place. You may be feeling anxious for example, asking yourself questions like; 'are the drugs working?', 'what effects are they going to have on my body or long-term health?', 'how am I going to cope with the side effects?'

Depression can set in as the drugs start to work on the cancer. Side effects, especially hair loss and tiredness which are caused by some of the drugs, can make you feel less good about your appearance. Having to change your normal routine to make time for the treatments can also be upsetting. Sometimes, if the cancer is taking time to respond to the drugs, you can start to become discouraged and feel depressed.

The greatest fear of all is fear of the unknown. Many cancer patients feel afraid of the future and what it might bring. Some also do not understand what is happening to their bodies and are frightened of the possible effects of the disease or the treatment.

How you can help yourself

Once you have identified why you are feeling as you are, you can start to take action to combat any negative emotions. Knowledge is an antidote to fear, so if you don't understand something about your treatment or disease or you want to know about side effects and possible outcomes of treatment – ask. If you don't understand the explanation, then keep asking until you do. Remember it is your right to know what is happening to your body and how your life may be affected. Most doctors and nurses are very willing to answer any questions and to keep you up-to-date on your progress.

Your emotional well-being is as important as your physical health. Everyone needs some support during difficult times and having cancer is one of the most stressful situations you are ever likely to face. If you feel that low moods are getting the better of you, try to talk over your feelings with some -one you feel close to and who can be a good listener. You may also find it helpful to discuss your feelings with a professional counsellor, a leader or member of your religious faith or a social worker. If you feel comfortable discussing personal worries with your doctor or nurse, then these people are often very good at helping you to bring your feelings out into the open and they can refer you to a trained counsellor or social worker for further help.

Of course, not all patients feel frightened or depressed during their treatment. There are ways in which you can smooth the course of your chemotherapy treatment.

The main aim should be to keep a positive attitude. To achieve this easy-to-say, difficult-to-do feat you need to know what your treatment involves, what is expected to happen, what side effects, if any, to expect, what can be done about them and what should be reported to your doctor. In short, you need to gather as much information as possible about your disease and treatment so you can play an active part in tackling your disease. Learning is an on-going process. You may need to ask questions over and over again or ask new questions every time you see your doctor. This is fine. It's your disease and you need to work with your doctor in order to beat it.

Regular updates on your progress are important for your emotional health. Asking your doctor for these will also give him or her an opportunity to reassure you if things are progressing rather more slowly than expected and to discuss changing your drugs or treatment plan if necessary.

Some people find it helpful to keep a diary or journal of their treatment. This can have several practical uses as well as providing an outlet for pent-up emotions. For example, you can record each time you felt sick and look back over your treatment to see how this fits in with your drugs. Changes to lessen side effects can often be made using information like this.

Writing down your thoughts can also help you to clarify any questions you may have for your doctor or nurse – and can help you to remember to ask them!

As your journal develops, you may find it encouraging to look back at how you coped during early low patches. Many people draw strength from realising that they came through before and can then believe they will do so again.

A private diary also allows you to 'say' anything that may be difficult for you to voice to someone else. Sometimes this can be used to prepare you to speak to a person about a problem or it can be used as a safety valve for anger or sadness that you feel you cannot express any other way.

Doing things for yourself will help you to feel more in control of your disease and treatment. You might like to look into learning relaxation or meditation techniques – the BACUP nurses can provide further information on these. Try to plan your time so you can still do the things that are most important to you. Although you should try not to let chemotherapy rob you of your social life, don't be too tough on yourself. Realistic goals are more likely to be achieved and are therefore better for your self-esteem. Taking some exercise – as long as it's not too strenuous – will raise your spirits and can help to get rid of tension. It is best to check with your doctor, however, before starting any new exercise programme.

How others can help you

Although there may be times when you want to be alone with your thoughts, at other times being able to share your feelings can be a weight off your mind. Patient support groups will put you in touch with other people undergoing similar treatment. Talking with these people can be a good way of giving vent to feelings relatives or friends may not understand and you can also pick up some useful 'coping tips'. BACUP can give you the addresses of your local support groups.

Family and friends usually want to help you bear the burden of coping. They may, however, find it difficult at first to grasp exactly what it is you are going through. The key is to keep communication going. Just at a time when you think loved ones should be rushing to your aid, they may stand back and wait for you to make the first move. This is often because they are worried they may say the wrong thing, or they think you may want to cope alone or they may even be feeling emotionally worn out themselves. Be open and honest about how your treatment is going and how you feel about it. In that way misunderstandings can be avoided and others are given opportunities to show their love and support.

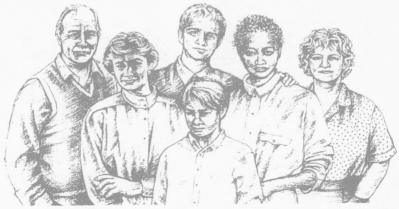

BACUP's cancer information service was set up to give you and your family information on all aspects of cancer and its treatment as well as on the practical and emotional problems of living with the illness. Information has been put together on computer about services available to cancer patients, research and treatment centres, cancer support groups, therapists and counsellors, financial assistance and home nursing services. Some of these are listed on the next few pages.

People often ring the service with queries about getting a mortgage or insurance after they have been diagnosed with cancer. BACUP has details of companies which specialise in these services.

If you would like any other booklets or help, you can ring and speak to one of our experienced cancer nurses. The service is open from 10am until 7pm Monday to Thursday and until 5.30pm on Friday.

If you are outside London you can call the service free of charge on 0800 181199. If you live within the London telephone area, you should call 071-608 1661.

Many people feel that counselling can help them deal with the problems of living with cancer. Counsellors use their skills to help people talk through and sort out some problem, difficulty or confusion. Emotional difficulties linked to cancer are not always easy to talk about and are often hardest to share with those to whom you are closest. Talking with a trained counsellor who is not personally involved can help to untangle thoughts, feelings and ideas.

BACUP's Cancer Counselling Service can give information about local counselling services and can discuss with people whether counselling could be appropriate and helpful for them. BACUP runs a one to one counselling service based at its London offices, which it is intended to develop nationwide.

For more information about counselling, or to make an appointment with BACUP's counselling service, please ring 071-608 1038 between 9am and 5.30pm.

Research — clinical trials

R esearch into new ways of using chemotherapy to treat cancer is going on all the time. As no current single drug or combination of drugs being used results in the cure of all patients treated, cancer doctors (oncologists) are continually looking for new drugs or combinations to treat the disease and they do this by using clinical trials.

Clinical trials are done to find out how effective a new drug is or whether it has fewer side effects than drugs which are equally effective. Patients take part in different phases of a trial depending on their general health, the type of cancer they have and how far it has spread, if at all. The trials are conducted in a way which ensures the patient has the highest standard of care.

Initially new drugs will have been well researched in laboratory tests, but the safest and most effective way of giving them will not yet have been tested on patients. People whose cancer will not be helped by any other treatment are offered very new drugs and doctors watch the patients very carefully for any beneficial or harmful effects of the drugs.

If these early trials show the drugs may be given safely, then further trials are done to test exactly how effective the drugs are against individual cancers.

If, at the end of these trials, the drugs seem to be as effective or more effective than current treatment, or they seem to have fewer side effects, they are tested in what is called a "controlled clinical trial". These trials directly compare the drugs under trial with the best current treatment to see which is the most effective. Many patients take part in these trials.

Usually, several hospitals around the country are involved in these trials. Your doctor, however, must have your informed consent before entering you into any phase of a clinical trial. This means that you know what the trial is about, you understand why it is being conducted and why you have been invited to take part, and you appreciate exactly how you will be involved.

In these trials, so that the treatments may be accurately compared, the type of treatment a patient receives is decided at random and not by the doctor treating the patient. This is because it has been shown that if a doctor chooses the treatment, or offers a choice to the patient, he or she may unintentionally bias the result of the trial.

Half the patients, therefore, will receive the best current treatment and the other half will receive the new treatment, which may or may not prove to be better than the current treatment.

If you agree to take part in a trial, you can still withdraw at any stage if you change your mind. Your decision will in no way affect your doctor's attitude towards you. If you choose not to take part or you withdraw from a trial, you will then receive the best current treatment rather than the new one with which it is being compared.

The reason why your doctor may want you to take part in a trial, is because until the new treatment has been tested scientifically in this way, it is impossible for doctors to know which is the best one to choose for their patients.

If you do choose to take part in these trials, it is important to remember that whatever treatment you receive will have been carefully researched in preliminary studies, before it is fully tested in any phase of a clinical trial. By taking part in a trial you will also be helping to advance medical science and thus improve prospects for patients in the future and it might benefit you.

Other Useful Organisations

CancerLink
17 Britannia Street
London WC1X 9JN
Tel: 071 833 2451

Resource centre for cancer self help and support groups throughout Britain and a telephone information service on all aspects of cancer.

Cancer Aftercare and Rehabilitation Society (CARE)
21 Zetland Road
Redland
Bristol BS6 7AH
Tel: 0272 427419

An organisation of cancer patients, relatives and friends who offer help and support. Branches throughout the country.

Cancer Relief Macmillan Fund
15-19 Britten Street
London SW3 3TY
Tel: 071 351 7811

Provides home care nurses through the Macmillan Service and financial grants for people with cancer and their families.

Marie Curie Cancer Care
28 Belgrave Square
London SW1X 8QG
Tel: 071 235 3325

*Runs eleven nursing homes throughout the UK and a
community nursing service to give extended care to patients
at home.*

Tak Tent
4th Floor
G Block
Western Infirmary
Glasgow G11 6NT
Tel: 041 332 3639

*Provides information, support and counselling for cancer
patients, their relatives and professional staff involved in their
care. Speakers are available for those interested in hearing
about the work of Tak Tent.*

Tenovus Cancer Information Centre
142 Whitchurch Road
Cardiff CF4 3NA
Tel: 0222 619846

*Provides a counselling and information service personally or
over the 'phone.*

The Ulster Cancer Foundation
40-42 Eglantine Avenue
Belfast BT9 6DX
Tel: 0232 663281

*Provides information over the 'phone about all aspects of
cancer.*

Recommended Reading List

Clyne, Rachael
Cancer Your Life, Your Choice
Wellingborough, Thorsons Publishing Group, 1989
(ISBN 0-7225-21-030)

Smedley, H, Sikora, K, and Stepney, R
Cancer: What it is and how it is treated
Oxford, Basil Blackwell, 1986
(ISBN 0-631-14041-7)

'Which' guide
Understanding Cancer
London, Consumers Association Publishers, 1986
(ISBN 0-340-37220-6)

Williams, Chris and Sue
Cancer: A guide for patients and their families
Chichester, Wiley, 1986
(ISBN 0-471-91017-1)

Bryan, Jenny, Lyall, Joanna
Living With Cancer
Penguin, 1987
(ISBN 0-14-009409-1)

Publications Available from BACUP

Coping with Hair Loss
Diet and the Cancer Patient
Chemotherapy
Radiotherapy
Acute Lymphoblastic Leukaemia
Acute Myeloblastic Leukaemia
Cancer of the Bladder
Cancer of the Bone
Brain Tumours
Cancer of the Breast
Cervical Smears
Cancer of the Cervix
Cancer of the Colon and Rectum
Chronic Lymphocytic Leukaemia
Chronic Myeloid Leukaemia
Hodgkins Disease
Cancer of the Kidney
Cancer of the Larynx

Cancer of the Liver
Cancer of the Lung
Malignant Melanoma
Myeloma
Non-Hodgkin's Lymphoma
Cancer of the Oesophagus
Cancer of the Ovary
Cancer of the Pancreas
Cancer of the Prostate
Cancer of the Skin
Cancer of the Stomach
Soft Tissue Sarcomas
Testicular Cancer
Cancer of the Thyroid
Cancer of the Uterus
Cancer of the Vulva
Cancer of the Mouth and
  Throat

For further information please contact:

BACUP
121-123 Charterhouse Street,
London, EC1M 6AA

Cancer Information Service 071 608 1661
Freeline (from outside London) 0800 181199
Administration 071 608 1785
Counselling Service 071 608 1038 (London-based)

BACUP's Cancer Information Service relies on voluntary
contributions to maintain its services. We need your help. If
you are interested in raising funds for BACUP, becoming a
'Friend' or helping in any other way please contact us.

Typeset and printed in Great Britain by Lithoflow Ltd, London